Skin Lesions and Wounds:

Burns, Cuts, Shingles, Skin Cancers and Pressure Ulcers

(Concepts, Causes, Diagnoses, Treatments and Care)

Solomon Barroa R.N.

To Dr. Lee Robbins, Mary Ann, Rosario, Vicente, Benedicto and Robert.

Foreword

Skin wounds and lesions occur to most of us as accidents. No one would want a skin wound or a lesion for life. It threatens our sense of safety and makes us anxious about what will happen to us next. Health information is essential for understanding and knowing what to say or do about these skin conditions. Such information can be acquired through the internet and conversations with healthcare professionals. These conversations often alleviate anxiety and uncertainty. The drawback with such conversation is the usage of medical terminologies. A non-medical person will not understand these medical terminologies resulting in ineffective disease management.

Chapter 1 talks about the anatomy and physiology of the skin. Our entire body is covered with skin. It protects us from the harsh environment that we live in. There are three layers of the skin: epidermis, dermis and subcutaneous tissue. This chapter will provide readers with the basic facts about the skin, it's functions and structures.

Chapter 2 is about skin integrity. The skin is also known as the integumentary system. Maintaining it's integrity is essential to keep a person's physical appearance at its best. Factors such as diseases and chemical substances pose a threat to the integrity of the skin. This chapter will provide the reader an understanding about skin integrity and how to keep it healthy.

Chapter 3 talks about the different types of skin lesions and wounds. Sometime in a person's life, a skin lesion has occurred. He or she may not know what it is and what to call it. Certain types of wounds and lesions impose risks to a person's well being. Examples of skin lesions are macules, papules, pustules, vesicles and nodules. Skin wounds exemplify abrasions and lacerations. This chapter will provide readers with basic knowledge about the different types of skin wounds and lesions.

Chapter 4 is about wound healing. The healing of a wound has different types and stages. The stages are inflammatory, migratory, proliferative and maturational. When a wound is healing, it is usually vulnerable to injury and infection. An understanding about the process of wound healing will enable the reader to accelerate the recovery.

Chapter 5 talks about skin cuts. Working in the kitchen predisposes a person to a skin cut. When it happens, interventions and treatment are needed and helpful. The initial intervention is to stop the bleeding by applying pressure. After the bleeding has stopped, placing a non-adherent dressing (depending on the degree of the skin cut) is the next step. This chapter will walk the reader through the process of wound care and treatment.

Chapter 6 is about skin cancer. The presence of skin cancer produces malignant skin lesion. There are three types of skin cancer: melanoma, squamous cell carcinoma and basal cell carcinoma. Their causes, diagnosis and treatment are discussed. This chapter will enable the reader to understand the concepts and treatment of skin cancer.

Chapter 7 talks about shingles. The varicella virus is the causative agent of shingles. It produces skin lesions composed of blisters that follow the nerve pathways. The pain is excruciating in a shingles infection. This chapter will provide the reader with knowledge about the mechanism or pathophysiology and treatment of shingles disease.

Chapter 8 is about pressure ulcers. Immobility is the number one cause of pressure ulcer among older adults. Recovery takes a long time because of the degenerative changes that occurs with aging. Stage 4 of a pressure ulcer extends to the muscles and bones. This can be prevented from happening with health education. This chapter will provide the reader with knowledge regarding the causes, types, treatments and care of pressure ulcer.

Chapter 9 talks about burns. An extensive burn is disfiguring if not unsettling. Skin grafts may be used to cover up the part of the skin that was extensively burned. There are instances when skin regeneration is effective and other forms of treatment may not be needed. The types, treatments and mechanism of the burn episode (pathophysiology) are discussed in this chapter providing the reader with a broad knowledge about burns.

Table Of Contents

Chapter 1 Anatomy and Physiology of the Skin   9

The Skin   9

Composition of the Skin   9

Structures of the Skin   10

Functions of the Skin   10

Skin Color   11

Chapter 2 Skin Integrity   12

Factors Affecting The Overall Integrity Of The Skin   12

Various Skin Conditions Affecting the Integrity Of The Skin   13

Chapter 3 Skin Lesions and Skin Wounds   15

Types of Skin Lesions   15

Types of Skin Wounds   16

Chapter 4 Wound Healing   17

Types of Wound Healing   17

Healing in Minor Wounds   17

Stages of Wound Healing   17

Scar Formation   18

Chapter 5 Skin Wounds : Intervention, Treatment, Care and Recovery   **19**

A Minor Skin Cut   19

A Deep Cut Wound and Its Intervention and Treatment   20

Caring and Recovering from Skin Wounds   21

Wound Care Equipment   22

Wound Care Procedure   23

Healing and Recovery   24

Chapter 6 Skin Cancer Lesions : Intervention, Treatment, Care and Recovery   **25**

Skin Cancer   25

Causes of Skin Cancer   25

Skin Cancer Prevention *26*

Types of Skin Cancer *26*

Basal Cell Carcinoma *26*

Squamous Cell Carcinoma *27*

Melanoma *27*

Intervention and Treatment for Skin Cancer *27*

Assessing for Skin Lesion *27*

Diagnosing Skin Cancer *28*

Caring and Recovering after a Skin Biopsy *28*

Treatment for Skin Cancer *28*

Caring and Recovering after Surgery, Chemotherapy and Radiation *29*

Chapter 7 Shingles Lesions: Intervention, Treatment, Care and Recovery **31**

Shingles *31*

The Mechanism of Shingles *31*

Intervention and Treatment of Shingles *32*

Caring and Recovering after Shingles *32*

Chapter 8 Pressure Ulcer Lesions and Wounds: Intervention, Treatment, Care and Recovery **33**

Pressure Ulcer *33*

Causative Factors of Pressure Ulcer *33*

Stages of Pressure Ulcer *34*

Stage 1 *35*

Stage 2 *35*

Stage 3 *35*

Stage 4 *35*

Intervention and Treatment for the Stages of Pressure Ulcer *36*

Care and Recovery from Pressure Ulcer *37*

Chapter 9 : Burn Lesions and Wounds: Intervention, Treatment, Care and Recovery **38**

Burns *38*

Causes of Burns *38*

Types of Burn According to the Area Involved *39*

First Degree Burns   *39*

Second Degree Burns   *39*

Third Degree Burns   *39*

Fourth Degree Burns   *39*

Bodily Response During a Burn Episode / Pathophysiology of Burns   *40*

Interventions and Treatment   *41*

Care and Recovery After A Burn Episode   *41*

Glossary   **42**

References   **44**

Index   **45**

Chapter 1 Anatomy and Physiology of the Skin

The Skin

The skin is the structure of the human body that is readily seen by the naked eye. It is composed of cells that maintain its unique appearance. The skin is also called the integumentary system. It comprises the external surface of the entire human body and is distributed from the head to the tip of the toe. It is about 16 % of our total body weight. Throughout the body, the skin of the palms and fingers are the thickest. Structures such as the hairs and nails complete the physical appearance of the human body. Melanin, a pigment produced by melanocytes, produces the skin color.

Composition of the Skin

The skin is made up of several layers. The outermost layer is the epidermis. It is comprised of five layers. Stratum corneum is the outermost layer that is seen by the naked eye. It consists mostly of keratin. This is also the place where bacteria and microorganisms thrive. It is always in contact with the outside world. Stratum lucidum comes next as the second layer. This layer is translucent. It acts as a barrier against bacterial invasion when the first layer gets injured. The third layer is comprised of stratum granulosum. This layer is granular in its characteristic. The stratum spinosum is the fourth layer. It is spinous in its characteristic due to its connectivity with other cellular elements such as lipids. This layer provides further protection from any type of skin injury. Stratum basale is the bottom layer that is connected to the dermis. This layer is germinative in its characteristic because of its ability to regenerate new cells. Stratum basale is also the layer where tactile receptors are situated. The most common bacteria in the epidermal layer of the skin is Staphylococcus Aureus. This bacteria can kill the person with a compromised immune system. Thus taking showers and washing hands are important regular safety practices for a healthy lifestyle.

The second layer of the skin is the dermis. It is not seen by the naked eye except when wounds occur. This is where blood vessels, lymphatic vessels, glands, nerves, sensory receptors and hair follicles are situated. When a skin wound occurs, the sensory nerves send signals to the brain to register pain. The blood vessels expel blood when the connection is broken. A series of reaction follow to stabilize the injured area of the skin. The third layer of the skin is the hypodermis mainly consisting of fatty tissues. This can be seen in the third stage of pressure ulcers and in deep wounds. When a deep wound occurs, a longer period of time may be needed for healing and recovery. This is true for some people like the older adults.

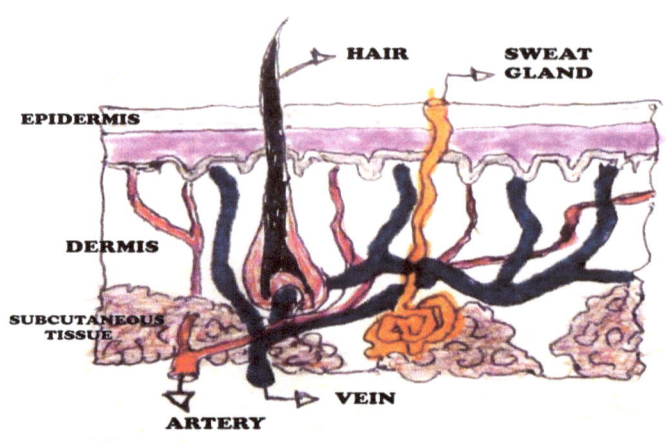

Layers and Structures of the Skin

Structures of the Skin

The accessory structures of the skin are hairs, glands and nails. Hair is the crowning glory on top of the head and present on almost all skin surfaces. The only exceptions are the palms and plantar area of the feet. Microbes like to live in hairy areas, and that is why shampooing the head and soaping body areas help to wash them away. Shaving the skin may improve appearance but any accidental cut can create a portal of entry for most microbes. The glands of the skin are composed of sebaceous sweat glands. These glands help in temperature regulation and production of sebum or oil that keeps moisture in the skin. It also helps to excrete urea and ammonia that causes body odor if present in profuse quantity. Nails are hardened plates that are keratinized. They serve to protect the toes and fingernails.

Functions of the Skin

The skin regulates body temperature due mainly to the sweat glands. In a heated environment, these glands produce sweat that is evaporated in the air causing a decrease in body temperature. The skin gives protection to the entire body through resisting microbes, preventing chemical penetration, heat insulation and abrasion. The skin also provides tactile sensations including touch, pressure, vibration, and thermal changes due to the nerve endings and receptors. Furthermore, the skin aids in excretion of salts, carbon dioxide, ammonia and urea through sweating. This is the reason why sweat is salty.

Finally, the skin also aids in absorption of certain drugs such as those contained in skin patches, gases, toxic chemicals (like that of carbon tetrachloride in some cleaning fluids), arsenic, lead, mercury and toxins in some poisonous plants known as the poison ivy. Thus, while the skin protects, it can also provide a channel for entry of damaging substances.

Skin Color

Skin color is due to the pigment melanin. This pigment is produced by the melanocyte cell. Varying amounts of melanin produce varying degrees of skin coloration from one person to another. A light skinned person has little melanin. Sunlight exposure tends to stimulate more of its production causing a tan appearance. Overexposure to sunlight eventually leads to skin cancer for some individuals. Always use sun protection.

The pigments carotene and hemoglobin also contribute to skin color. Hemoglobin pigment produces a pinkish to reddish appearance of the skin. The yellowish appearance of the skin is not due to any skin pigment but rather is a symptom of a disease such as viral hepatitis.

Chapter 2 Skin Integrity

Factors Affecting The Overall Integrity Of The Skin

There are many factors that promote a healthy looking skin. One of these is the nutritional intake of a person. Eating a balanced diet with antioxidants, vitamins A, C, and E, zinc and selenium leads to a healthy skin. Most of these nutrients are found in everyday foods such as broccoli, carrots, almonds, kiwi, oranges and many others. Supplements are readily available to compensate for a deficient intake.

Another factor is adequate hydration. Drinking at least 8 glasses of water will enable blood circulation and hydration of skin cells. Hygienic practices as described earlier, wash away microbes and generally cleanse the skin. If showers are not possible on a daily basis, at least every other day is essential to prevent build up of body dirt and odor. Use a mild or hypoallergenic soap, either liquid or bar, to avoid irritation and loss of body oils.

Bodily conditions such as blood clots can lead to inadequate systemic blood circulation to the skin. Skin breakdown eventually occurs. Blood circulation has two types: systemic and local. Systemic blood circulation affects the overall skin integrity. Local blood circulation on the other hand is limited to certain parts of the skin.

Mobility and exercises promote blood circulation to the skin. An immobile and bed ridden person will be susceptible to skin pressure leading to ulcers. It is important to ambulate whenever possible. If it isn't possible to do so, perform range of motion exercises and change positions in bed to promote blood circulation.

Strong chemicals from cosmetics and agents used either temporarily or to remove unwanted facial structures are another factor in skin integrity. These agents exfoliate the top layers of the skin. With the exfoliation, deep shedding of the epidermis occurs. In some instances these agents create facial discoloration. A person should do research regarding the chemical ingredients of cosmetics sold over the counter before using them. If in doubt speak to a dermatologist or a skin specialist. Seeking the help of a skin professional to improve facial skin is often the best choice.

Too much skin exposure to the sun presents itself as a crucial factor in causing difficulty in maintaining overall skin integrity. Such excessive exposure predisposes a person to both precancerous and cancerous lesions, mottled pigmentation, freckles and rapid aging. Eventually, the fibers of the skin called elastin are damaged by the sun causing less stretchability and elasticity.

Emotions also play a role in the integrity of the skin. The different systems in the body including the skin, are interdependent with each other. Stress that occurs anywhere at anytime induces an emotional reaction. Anything emotional produces chemical reactions inside the body as chemical substances trigger a response. Moderate to severe emotional stress for instance, causes the sebaceous glands to produce more oil resulting in acne.

Using household chemicals to clean the kitchen and other parts of the house without hand gloves can also damage the skin. Strong chemicals such as carbon tetrachloride in cleaning fluids will slough off some of the epidermal layers. Always use hand gloves whenever handling such strong chemicals. Wash the hands with mild or hypoallergenic soap following use of such chemicals.

Finally, sleep relaxes and promotes the development of skin cells. This is the period where skin cell renewal primarily occurs. Insomnia and lack of sleep produces dull looking skin. The recommended hours for sleeping are from 6 – 9 to promote regular circadian rhythm in a 24 hour.

Various Skin Conditions Affecting the Integrity Of The Skin

Skin integrity can be defined as the over all health and functionality of the skin and its structures. There are numerous problematical skin conditions that affect the integrity of the skin. Such skin conditions have causative factors. Microbes, sharp objects and bodily diseases play a role in the existence of such skin conditions. The integrity of the skin is threatened and often impaired by these factors.

Cellulitis, shingles, cancer, burns, pressure ulcer and inflammatory conditions can locally impair the skin integrity. Cellulitis is an infection of the deep layers of the dermis. It is caused by the bacteria staphylococcus that is acquired through a wound. Symptoms will be swelling, redness, pain and itching. The treatment of choice is antibiotics. Shingles or Herpes Zoster is an acute viral infection of the peripheral nerve pathways. It is caused by the varicella zoster virus. It occurs in people who have had chickenpox or are immune compromised by chemotherapy and HIV. The presenting symptoms of shingles are pain, itching and formation of vesicles that follow the nerve pathways. Shingles is treated with an antiviral drug called acyclovir.

Skin cancer is a cellular aberration on top of the skin that may extend to the dermis. It can spread rapidly through metastasis. Skin cancer is initially asymptomatic. There will be changes in the color and size of the lesion when it becomes malignant. It can be treated with surgery, chemotherapy and radiation. Skin cancer is readily curable if detected in the early stages.

Skin burns are wounds and ulcerations of the skin. They are caused by chemical, electrical, thermal and radiation agents. The burn can be systemic or localized in occurrence. Burns produces cellular destruction and depletion of both fluids and electrolytes. The course of treatment is not an easy task as it consists of debridement, administration of antibiotics, grafting and other methods.

Pressure ulcer is the result of applying strong pressure on the skin over a period of time. It eventually causes an occlusion of blood circulation in the affected areas. Pressure ulcers occurs most frequently at bony prominences. It produces tissue damage, erythema,

pain, loss of sensation and other symptoms depending on its stage. Extensive treatment with debridement, dressing, supplementation and antibiotics is necessary.
Inflammatory skin conditions such as seborrheic dermatitis, eczema, intertrigo and psoriasis also compromises the integrity of the skin. Symptoms such as swelling, itchiness, scales and dryness of the skin are some of the symptoms presented. These symptoms are treated accordingly.

Acne vulgaris is a multi factorial disorder. Its exact cause is unknown. The symptoms of acne are lesions comprising of comedones (open and closed), pustules, papules and nodules. The treatment of choice is application of benzoyl peroxide to the affected skin.

Chapter 3 Skin Lesions and Skin Wounds

Types of Skin Lesions

A skin lesion can be defined in various ways. It is an abnormal growth or patch in the skin, either acquired congenitally or as a result of a disease condition and skin trauma. A lesion can turn into a wound or remain as a lesion until it is removed or treated. Skin lesions not only threaten the integrity of the skin but it also create an unsightly appearance for some people. The removal of skin lesions has been a part of the cosmetic industry and has been revolutionized in today's day and age.

There are different types of skin lesions such as macules, papules, nodules, moles, tumors, wheals, vesicles, bulla, pustules, plaques, fissures, erosions, ulcers, crusts and scales. A macule is a flat, circumscribed and non-elevated skin structure. It can measure from 1 centimeter or higher. Freckles and flat moles are examples of macules. Papules are raised and circumscribed skin structures. Warts are examples of papules. A nodule is a raised solid skin structure that extends inward to the dermis. A mole or a pigmented nevi is an example of a nodule. Tumors are raised solid skin structures extending to the dermis that usually exceed 2 cm. Dermatofibroma is an example of a tumor. A wheal is a flattened fluid-filled skin structure measuring from 1 mm to several centimeters. Mosquito bites and skin testing reaction are good examples of wheals. Vesicles are raised fluid filled skin structures, usually less than 5 mm in size. Common occurrences of vesicles arise in the illness of shingles that is caused by the herpes zoster virus. It occurs particularly among elderly people and in those subject to high levels of stress.

A bulla is a fluid filled skin structure of over 1 cm in size. Second degree burns resembles a bulla. Pustules are fluid filled skin structures with pus over 1 cm in size such as those found in boils and acne. A plaque is a bright red colored and scaly to silvery skin structure. Psoriasis skin infection contains skin plaques. Fissures are cracks in the skin.

Athlete's foot is a good example of a fissure. An erosion is a loss of superficial dermis. It is usually without the presence of blood just like when the lesion of chickenpox ruptures. Ulcers are deep losses of the skin surface resembling that of a pressure ulcer. A crust is a dried residue from blood or pus. An impetigo skin condition contains a lot of crusts. Scales are flakes of exfoliated epidermis. Dandruffs are examples of scales consisting of exfoliated dermis.

Types of Skin Wounds

A skin wound is defined as a condition where there is a break in the continuity of the skin. It can extend pass the hypodermis and into the muscles. Skin wounds can be classified in different ways; open, closed, superficial and penetrating. This book will limit the examples to open wounds since it focuses on skin.

The common types of skin wounds are abrasions, lacerations, skin cuts and punctures. An abrasion is a scraping of the skin due to rubbing and friction from rough surfaces. Examples are a skinned knee from a fall and skin scraping from a shoe. Laceration is the tearing of the skin and tissues due to a strong force. It is characterized by jagged and uneven edges. A large baby passing through the birth canal causes vaginal tears and laceration of adjacent tissues. Skin cut is any slicing in the continuity of the skin. Knife cuts in the kitchen and paper cuts in the office are examples. Punctures are narrow but deep skin wounds. Needle injections among drug addicted persons produce puncture wounds.

Closed wounds on the other hand do not break the skin integrity where internal organs and tissues are involved. It may predispose an affected person to internal bleeding. In most cases bruising, pain and swelling present as the major symptoms. There are also cases when symptoms occur after a week or so. A typical example of a closed wound is trauma to the head during a fight.

Chapter 4 Wound Healing

Types of Wound Healing

Wound healing is a process wherein new tissue is generated to replace the damaged one. It occurs in several stages. Time, patience and care are the main considerations in promoting wound healing. Factors affecting the healing process are discussed in the next chapter.

There are three types of wound healing termed healing by first intention, by second intention and by third intention. Healing by first intention is faster and simplest. Wound edges are attached together either by suture or stitches, staples or bandages. Healing by second intention is slower because of the drainage from an infection, and it usually involves a much larger wounded area. The wound in second intention is usually filled with fragile granulation tissue. Healing by third intention is the slowest. It can take a longer period of time such as a month before it heals. As per physicians' order, the wound is observed before closing it. A skin graft may be applied to enhance the appearance.

Healing in Minor Wounds

Skin wound such as an abrasion involves only the epidermis of the skin. This kind of wound heals very fast. Examples are abrasion from an object such as a shoe and from accidental falling. The epidermis has basal cells that migrate across the wound. The migration stops because of a cellular response that causes contact inhibition. During the migration process, a hormone called epidermal growth factor stimulates basal cells to replace the damaged cells constructing a structure that thickens to form a new epidermis.

Stages of Wound Healing

In deep large wounds, there are 4 stages of healing; inflammatory, migratory, proliferative and maturation. Initially there is an inflammatory phase, which lasts about 3 days. In this phase blood components such as the white blood cells engulf bacteria through phagocytosis, clotting factors form blood clots and histamines are released resulting in vasodilation and exudation. The inflammatory phase causes localized redness, edema, warmth and some throbbing sensation. This phase may be prolonged by certain factors such as malnutrition and lifestyle habits as discussed in the next chapter.

The migratory phase which takes 3– 5 days comes after the inflammation phase. In this phase, fibroblasts cells migrate to the newly formed blood clot and begin synthesizing collagen fibers in the dermis. With the presence of collagen, a granulation tissue emerges. Collagen is the main component of a scar tissue. It provides structure to the wound.

Proliferative phase is the third stage of wound healing. It requires approximately 5 – 24 days varying in duration from person to person. In this phase tissues and blood vessels are formed. Epithelialization, wound contraction and further granulation also occur. The wound is reconstructed continuously in this last phase. Healing can be impaired due to malnutrition, age or an unhealthy lifestyle.

Last is the maturation phase. In this phase, granulation tissue in the dermis develops into scar tissue and continuously gains strength. This phase may take place from months to a year depending on the severity of damage to the wounded area. Nutritional status, age, and lifestyle habits are also factors that can affect this last phase of wound healing.

Scar Formation

Scars occur due to the granulation tissue formed during the maturational phase of healing. Sizes of scars will vary depending on the wounded area and the healing process. The scar tissue formation is also known as fibrosis. If a scar tissue extends beyond the boundaries of the wound, it is called a keloid. Hypertrophic scars, on the other hand, remain within boundaries of the wound. Scars are less elastic compared to normal skin. For psychological reasons, some people have their scars removed by a cosmetic surgeon. It may relieve them of a memory of their ordeal and makes the skin appear better. Some scars disappear as time passes due to the natural sloughing of skin cells.

Chapter 5 Skin Wounds : Intervention, Treatment, Care and Recovery

A Minor Skin Cut

Some people are quick and precise in responding to emergency situations. The sight of blood does not provoke fear, and measures to correct the situation are instantly performed. Such a person can work in an emergency room treating all types of skin wounds. In the occurrence of a minor skin cut, a person doesn't need a medical background to implement measures for relieving such a skin wound. The presence of open mindedness, concern for safety and well-being are tools for effective interventions. For some people who are fearful, dependency on medical personnel helps them pass through the ordeal. The emotional support and extensive knowledge of a physician and a nurse practitioner alleviate the anxiety of the wounded person as interventions are done to correct the condition.

For a minor superficial skin cut from a kitchen knife, we do not rush to the emergency room but rather we implement steps to stop the bleeding. Our instinct and often the lessons that we learned from our parents and significant others, consciously prompt us to apply pressure for 3 - 5 minutes to stop the bleeding and to use a simple band aid strip to cover the wound. Mild pain is felt from time to time as cells regenerate to stabilize the wound.

Signs and symptoms of infection can happen during a skin cut. These are swelling, presence of odorous and purulent drainage, fever, warmth, pain and tenderness on the wound site. If any of these occur, consult your medical care provider immediately. For some people who don't have health insurance, research and self-medication can be a helpful alternative. Some people would use alternative options such as herbs; some just ignore these more serious symptoms believing that they will fix themselves in due time. Self-medication is never the best option unless you are a doctor and knowledgeable about the drugs and method that you will be using. Certain herbs such as echinacea are used by other people for infection. They believe that these stimulate the immune system and have anti-inflammatory properties.

A Deep Cut Wound and Its Intervention and Treatment

A deep cut wound is a situation where there is more intense pain and blood is either oozing profusely or gushing out. There are two basic blood types that may be seen in any skin cut wound, arterial and venous. Arterial blood is bright red and spouts unevenly due to the pressure produced by the heart's outward pumping mechanism. It is bright red in color because it was already oxygenated in the lungs. Oxygenated blood is essential to the various cell, tissues, and organs of the body. Venous blood is dark maroon and flows evenly. It is a type of blood that has not been oxygenated in the lungs. It carries carbon dioxide instead of oxygen.

If you or someone you know had a deep cut, apply first aid initially to stop the bleeding. To do this, apply pressure for at least 5 minutes or more. The pressure depresses the skin edges of the wounded skin and partially connects it together. Apply direct pressure not with your bare hands but with a clean material such as a washcloth if no dressing is available. Wearing gloves is advisable if available as it prevents infection and contamination. Depending on the body part involved, elevating the wounded part higher than the heart while applying pressure helps to stop the bleeding.

In a home setting whenever the bleeding has stopped or even before it stops, calling help from a healthcare professional is a must. This healthcare professional may apply a non-adherent dressing on top of the wound depending on circumstances and wound assessment. In the event that there is no dressing available, a larger bandaid for a small deep cut and a clean and moist washcloth for longer deep wounds may be used. Wound care may differ depending on the equipment available at the time of the injury. Assessment of the wounded person for other physical symptoms related to blood loss is needed. Hypovolemic shock may happen because of excessive blood loss or hemorrhage. Look for signs of apprehension and restlessness, weakness of one or two extremities, sweating, cold skin and whether there is some loss of consciousness or lethargy. If several or most of these signs are manifested, call 911 immediately.

Blood will form a clot and will initially bind the separated parts of the skin. If bleeding doesn't stop with or without other symptoms such as weakness or dizziness, call 911 and report the current condition of the wounded person. Ambulance personnel will arrive to make their best effort to stabilize the bleeding and eventually the vital signs. The wounded person should be immediately transported to the emergency room.

Excessive blood loss or hemorrhage predisposes the wounded person to hypovolemic shock characterized by a decreased circulating blood volume. Upon arrival in the emergency room, a thorough assessment will be made by the nurse or even the admitting personnel.

When the bleeding subsides, a non-adherent dressing is taped over the skin wound which further allows skin edges to close and blood clots to form. In the event that the dressing is still soaked in blood, the nurse will add another layer of dressing and apply further pressure to stop the bleeding. Some skin wounds need immediate suturing by the physician on duty. In cases of animal bites, bleeding is allowed as it removes toxins and then the wound can be stabilized. For objects that penetrated the skin such as a knife, abrupt removal is avoided to prevent hemorrhage.

Caring and Recovering from Skin Wounds

After stabilizing the wound and applying non-adherent dressing to the wounded person, care and recovery is the next step. The objective is to avoid recurrence and aggravating what is already stable. Make sure that there are no signs of infection and hypovolemic shock. An infection can happen after several days due to poor care management and lack of knowledge about wound care.

In the hospital setting, a wounded person can be expected to receive the appropriate care. Upon discharge, a dressing will be in place and further instruction for wound care provided. In the event that caregivers are not able to perform wound care, a visiting nurse or a home health nurse can do it. Caring for a wound is not an easy task for the inexperienced. There are instances wherein a household member may take the responsibility for wound care.

Wound Care Equipment

The necessary equipment and medications for wound care should be in place such as hand gloves, non-adherent dressing or gauze pad to cover the wound size, antiseptic and cleansing solution as instructed by the physician, antibiotic solution as prescribed, kidney basin or a glass, forceps if needed, scissor and medical tape. This equipment can be bought at any pharmacy and make sure you have enough supply or even extras because some people have slow healing periods.

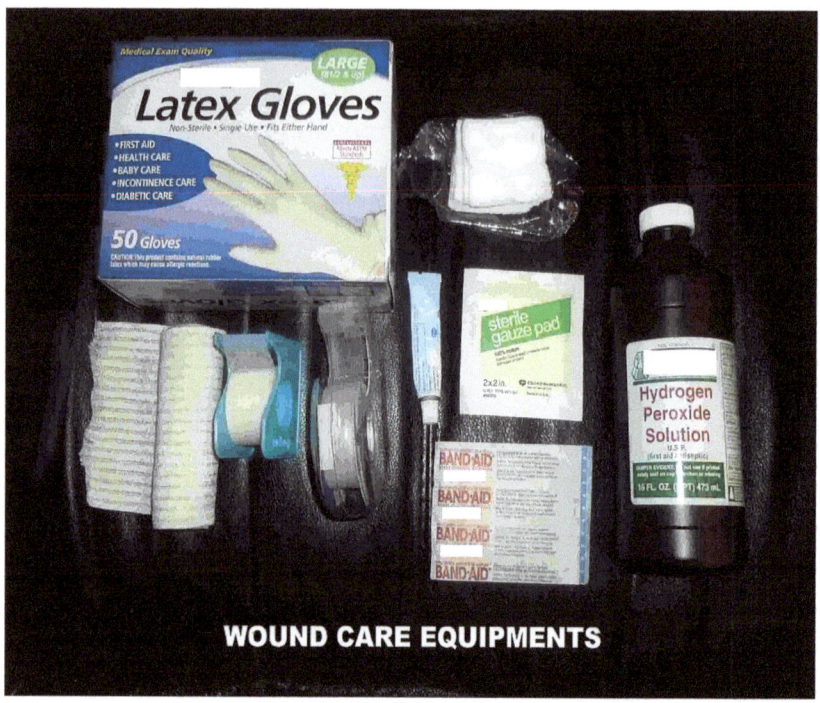

WOUND CARE EQUIPMENTS

Cleansing solution and antiseptic comes in various kinds. Normal saline is the safest because it doesn't have any inert chemical, and it is used to irrigate and clean the wound and its surrounding. Hydrogen peroxide is used as an oxidizing agent. It softens and removes crust and should not be used if there is a granular tissue, which is a part of the healing process. Povidone Iodine is an antibacterial and liberates at least 10 % iodine; critic says that it delays the healing process due to its toxicity. Acetic acid is an antibacterial used against Pseudomonas aeruginosa and may slow the healing period. Sodium hypochloride is an antimicrobial and effective against staphylococci and streptococci organisms. It is a tissue irritant and may delay the healing process. Regardless of whatever prescribed solution, always ask the physician about the pros and cons.

Wound dressings comes in two types, wet and dry. Dry dressing simply means application of dry dressing to a wound. Gauze dressing is commonly used because it causes little wound irritation. It comes in various sizes such as 10 x 10 cm or 5 x 5 cm. Wet dressings are used for wounds that will require debridement. Gauze is soaked in a cleansing solution and placed over the wound to remove crusts and debris. Hydrocolloid and hydrogel dressings such as Duoderm are occlusive. They absorb drainage through the use of exudate absorbers beneath the dressing, humidify wounds, liquefy debris and provides a protective cushion.

Telfa is an example of a non-adherent gauze as it doesn't stick to the wound but allows wound exudates and drainage to pass through to the softened gauze above it. A transparent film type of dressing can be used for smaller wounds as it permits viewing and adheres to the unwounded skin. Always ask the physician for more information.

Wound Care Procedure

The initial procedure is to talk to the wounded person, ask permission and explain what you want to do with the wound. Anybody can refuse treatment and care of their own will and volition. If this happens, find a good time of the day where the wounded person is comfortable to talk about wound care and possibly support them in self care. Continuously educate and motivate the wounded person about the importance of wound care.

Depending on the wounded persons' condition either bedridden or ambulatory, consider the most comfortable position and ensure privacy. Gather all necessary equipment. Begin wound care by washing your hands and putting on gloves that fit your size. The antiseptic solution is poured into a sterile basin or a glass. Place towels, or absorbent bed pads if bedridden, and drape if necessary to expose only the wounded part. Remove soiled dressing by detaching tape manually or use a solution to detach the tape to prevent pain and pressure. Pull the tape toward the dressing to reduce stress on the wound edges. Discard the soiled dressing in the trash bag. Observe the appearance of the wound and whether there are exudates and drainage. Check for signs of infection such as pus or green exudates; note if there is a granular tissue as a sign of healing, and observe if there is dehiscence or separation of wound layers. Notify the physician or primary healthcare provider immediately if there is a sign of infection or dehiscence. To begin cleaning the wound, soak gauze in the antiseptic solution and use forceps if present to pick up the moistened gauze. With the forceps or gloved hands, use gentle strokes to clean the wound from least contaminated to most contaminated areas of the wound. Then use dry gauze to finalize the cleaning process. All used gauze should be disposed in the trash bag. Apply prescribed antiseptic solution directly to the wound or as instructed by the physician. There are two ways of applying a gauze, wet or dry. It will depend on a physician's order and the outcome of the wound assessment. Apply either a dry or wet dressing after cleaning the wound and tape it. Remove your gloves and dispose of them in a trash bag.

In cases of wet to dry dressing, antiseptic ointment is usually omitted and a wet dressing is placed directly over the wound and dry dressing is placed on top of the wet dressing. Wound irrigation is also done in some cases. A syringe is filled with normal saline, and used to slowly flush the wound. Saline solution drains to the basin. The use of bandages and binders is done in some cases so as to immobilize a body part and support a wound.

Healing and Recovery

The healing process is affected by factors such as malnutrition, smoking or alcoholism, drugs, chronic diseases and aging. Malnutrition is the deficient intake of nutrients such as protein that aid in the healing process. Protein is considered the building block of the cell. It promotes growth of tissue. Collagen as a protein is needed by the fibroblasts cells and vitamin C is required for the synthesis of collagen. A well balanced diet consisting of protein, carbohydrates, lipids, vitamins and minerals is best. Smoking, alcoholism and drug addiction always interferes with normal cellular mechanisms. These types of habit decrease the amount of tissue oxygenation and lead to hypercoagulability. Prescribed drugs such as steroids will slow the inflammatory process and collagen synthesis.

Chemotherapeutic drugs can depress the development of leukocytes causing an impaired inflammatory response. Abuse of antibiotics predisposes the wounded person to super-infection as bacteria become resistant. Anti-inflammatory drugs suppress the synthesis of protein and the inflammation process. Chronic diseases such as diabetes mellitus can impede proper tissue oxygenation. Aging itself slows the healing process. An older adult has decreased bodily function in all aspects such as a reduced liver function, a decrease in antibody formation, a slowed inflammatory process, vascular changes that provide inadequate oxygenation to the wounded site, and a collagen and scar tissue that is not as pliable and elastic.

Infection can happen after stabilizing the wound or after application of a dressing. This delays or stops the healing process. Any unsterile object or ungloved hands that touches the wound directly will ultimately cause infection. Signs of infection are usually evident after 2 to 3 days. As mentioned earlier, signs of infection are swelling, pain, tenderness, odorous and purulent drainage, fever and warmth on the wound site. The physician will order a wound culture to determine the type of bacteria in the event of an infection. A wound culture also has a relationship to the color of the wound drainage.

Chapter 6 Skin Cancer Lesions : Intervention, Treatment, Care and Recovery

Skin Cancer

A skin cancer is a malignant lesion that grows steadily or can accelerate at some point. It presents itself on the surface of the skin with varying appearances such as in asymmetrical shapes and unequal sizes. It is usually an asymptomatic lesion except when metastasis occurs. Metastasis is the proliferation and outbreak of malignant cells from a specific location. It may spread to surrounding structures and travel through the blood stream. The symptoms of metastasis are bleeding, pain and changes in size and color. Skin cancer is most treatable when it is small. Prevention is achieved through an early diagnosis from a dermatologist. A skin sample is usually taken and analyzed in a laboratory. A diagnosis will be formulated after thorough analysis of the skin sample. Assessment and meticulous observation is the foundation for early treatment.

Causes of Skin Cancer

The most common cause of skin cancer is ultraviolet radiation from excessive sun exposure. The time of the day where sun rays are intense is believed to be from around 10 in the morning up to 4 in the afternoon. Exposure of the skin to toxic chemicals such as radium and arsenic compounds is also believed to cause skin cancer. These chemicals are used in some industrial plants with industrial workers exposed on a regular basis. Furthermore, tanning booths are believed to have caused skin cancer due to the ultraviolet exposure emitted from the machine. There are ways to tan oneself aside from using a tanning booth. Tanning skin sprays with non-toxic chemicals are used by some people to achieve a tannish look. Genetics may play a role in skin cancer development due to genetic coding transmitted from parent to offspring. The role of genes in skin cancer is still under investigation.

Skin Cancer Prevention

During sun exposure, use sun screen on any exposed areas. The current recommended sun protection factor for any sunscreen lotion is 15 and higher. It is recommended to reapply the lotion after two hours. The chemical ingredients titanium dioxide and zinc oxide are recommended by dermatologists. The tiny nano-particles of these substances, though still controversial, have the advantage of being invisible on the skin once rubbed in. These two chemical ingredients of sunscreen reflect and absorb the ultraviolet rays of the sun. They enable skin protection by coating and preserving the skin cells.

Limit exposure to the sun. If possible, avoid sun exposure from 10 am to 4 pm because ultraviolet radiation is at its strongest or highest level during these times. Wear a wide-brimmed hat and sunglasses whenever possible. Protective clothing is advisable to prevent sun rays from coming into contact with the skin. Light and transparent clothes will not do the job for sun protection; instead wear thicker ones with a tighter weave. An estimate of the clothing's effectiveness may be made by the layperson by simply looking through a layer of the fabric towards the sun and noting how much of the light is transmitted. In cases of tanning under the sun, issues arise because some people have a desire to get tanned. If it isn't possible to stop tanning, limiting and gradual exposure may be a harm reduction technique.

Avoid exposure to chemical irritants such as arsenic compound and carbon tetrachloride that are present in household cleaners. They are readily absorbed by the skin. These chemicals interact with the skin cells causing necrosis and permanent damage. Necrosis is a condition where cells and tissues die because of toxic conditions and the absence of nourishment. It is wise to always check the chemical consistency of a household product before using it at home or at the workplace.

Types of Skin Cancer

Basal Cell Carcinoma

Carcinoma is a cancer affecting the epithelial cells of any structure in the human body. The epithelial cells cover the surface of the different organs of the human body including the skin. This type of skin cancer is the most common and generally situated in the face. It is also seen in sun exposed areas such as the neck, arms and legs. Basal cell carcinoma arises from the epidermal structure of the skin. Metastasis is rare but trigger factors such as ultraviolet radiation can predispose its occurrence. It appears as a waxy nodule that is raised and pearly. There may be telangiectasis or dilated blood vessels. It is mostly translucent and bleeding will occur. It is likened to a sore that does not heal.

Squamous Cell Carcinoma

The squamous cell is another type of epithelial cell. In addition to the skin, it exists in different organs of the body such as the bladder and the lungs. Squamous cell carcinoma is a type of skin cancer that develops rapidly towards metastasis and can be a result of other precancerous lesions. It appears as a red, small, crusty and sometimes scaly patch on the skin. Ulceration and bleeding may occur at anytime. It arises in sun-exposed areas as does the basal cell carcinoma.

Melanoma

Melanoma is a skin cancer that arises from the melanocytes that produces the skin pigment. Melanin is the skin pigment that creates the skin color of a person. It is comprised of melanocytes. These melanocytes are located in the basal cells of the epidermis.

The appearance of melanoma is asymmetrical with irregular borders. Color varies but it is mostly black. Variations in color are brown, pink, gray, blue, red, white or a fleshy color. Melanoma is a very aggressive type of cancer and is malignant. It metastasizes rapidly to other organs of the body.

Intervention and Treatment for Skin Cancer

Assessing for Skin Lesion

Observing and assessing the skin lesion and mole on a regular basis is the initial step for detecting skin cancer. A person should undress and stand naked in front of the mirror to look for any existing skin lesion. The iris of the eye should also be checked for spots because skin cancer can occur there. If there is a lesion; note the color, size in terms of asymmetry and border irregularity, diameter, location and if there is pain or blood. Use a second hand mirror to look at the back or have a companion do so. If a day or week has passed and changes occurred, consult the primary care provider or a dermatologist immediately. Take precaution not to irritate the skin lesion.

A mole can sometimes be cancerous as it arises from skin pigmentation primarily that of melanin. Moles that are present at birth are generally not cancerous. If it appears after age 30, chances are that it will be cancerous. Observing the various moles of the body is recommended. Changes in the size, color, border and diameter of a mole signifies cellular activity. Consult a dermatologist immediately if such changes occur.

Diagnosing Skin Cancer

Upon arrival to the physician's office, a thorough assessment is done. Moles and skin lesions are inspected. A thorough assessment will be done and a skin biopsy will be ordered for a suspected lesion. Skin biopsy is a procedure where a skin sample is taken to determine what specific type of cell is involved. It also provides an analysis if skin cells are cancerous. There are different types of skin biopsy; shave, punch and excisional. Excisional biopsy is a procedure where the entire skin lesion is removed. A thorough sampling and removal of precancerous lesion is achieved in this procedure. A punch biopsy is a procedure where a circular blade is used to cut samples of a skin lesion. The remaining lesion is observed for physical changes. A shave biopsy is made possible by cutting sample of the skin. Regardless of the kind of biopsy, skin sample is sent to a laboratory. When it arrives, the skin sample is further cut and blended with a solution. Once this is done, it will be ready for viewing in a microscope. It will be stained again with a solution for being looked at in a microscope. With careful analysis, a determination will be done to formulate a diagnosis.

Caring and Recovering after a Skin Biopsy

To promote wound healing care should be taken not to irritate the skin lesion while waiting for the laboratory results. Avoid applying pressure on the skin lesion. The use of chemical irritants should also be avoided. Cover the skin lesion if sun exposure is unavoidable with a gauze pad placed on top of the excised lesion. Pain medications may be prescribed to alleviate painful sensations. Antibiotic solution may be prescribed to avoid infection. Instructions regarding changing gauze pad and cleaning the site will be provided by the health care provider. Observe the site for signs of infection such as bleeding, drainage or exudates, warmth and swelling. If such signs are observed, contact the primary care provider immediately. Usually a laboratory report is available in under a week.

Treatment for Skin Cancer

After the diagnosis of skin cancer is relayed to the client, options for treatment are discussed. Treatments for a skin cancer include surgery, chemotherapy, radiation and cryosurgery. Surgery entails removing the entire cancerous lesion and some of the surrounding tissue, which may include nearby lymph nodes to avoid recurrence. A skin graft is used to cover the surgical site if there is extensive excision.

Chemotherapy is a procedure that involves the administration of anti-cancer drugs known as chemotherapeutic agents. These drugs can be topical creams, drugs infused into the vein to produce systemic effect or orally administered drugs. Chemotherapeutic agents are used to prevent cancer cells from dividing to form another group of cancerous cells.

Chemotherapeutic creams such as fluorouracil and imiquimod can be used if the choice is topical chemotherapy. The common side effects of these creams are redness, itching and swelling. Intravenous cisplatin is usually prescribed if intravenous therapy is chosen. The common side effect is some gastrointestinal discomfort such as nausea, vomiting or diarrhea. The gastrointestinal area of the human body is the area where the stomach and intestines are located. The oral cavity also may acquire sores and ulcers.

Radiation therapy is another option. There are two specific types of radiation therapy; internal and external. External radiation involves the emission of radioactive light onto the skin cancer while internal radiation is the implantation of sealed radioactive substances in wires or seeds directly at the affected site. A side effect of radiation is often redness and blistering of the skin. A skin solution will be prescribed to relieve these symptoms.

There are newer methods of treating skin cancer such as cryosurgery. This procedure involves the use of liquid nitrogen to freeze the tumor. After the application of liquid nitrogen, the skin lesion is refrozen and allowed to thaw until it becomes somewhat gelatinous. The site become swollen and healing can require up to 6 weeks depending on the size of the tumor.

These are different ways of treating a skin cancer. The option for selecting an appropriate treatment requires considering its effect on the lifestyle of a patient. A treatment with less disruption and fewer side effects is usually chosen. A combination of either surgery or chemotherapy may be the better option to prevent the cancerous cell from recurring.

Caring and Recovering after Surgery, Chemotherapy and Radiation

Post-operative care will be a challenge for some people. Quality wound care such as changes in the surgical dressing will be implemented to avoid infection. Adherence to a prescribed treatment regimen is a must. Constant follow-up with the primary care provider is also necessary. Observing the operated site for signs of infection such as drainage and swelling, eating a well balanced diet to promote the healing process, avoiding pressure on the surgical site as well as exposure to chemical irritants are good care management techniques for a post operative incision.

While on chemotherapy, side effects will vary greatly depending on a persons' genetic makeup. Gastrointestinal discomfort may prevent a person from taking in sufficient nutrients. Consulting a dietician and nutritionist can be beneficial. Loss of hair can also happen which can have an impact on the self-perception and confidence of the person on chemotherapy. Rather than staying indoors all the time, a short walk in shady areas whlle wearing a hat provides a better alternative.

Radiation therapy has fewer side effects. One which does occur is skin irritation producing redness and swelling. Avoid sun exposure, use hypoallergenic products, wear non-constrictive clothing over the affected area, and never scrub it when washing with lukewarm water. Another effect of radiation is fatigue. Conserve energy by resting, performing less vigorous activities and asking help from other members of the household.

Regardless of a single method or a combination of treatments, recovery will depend on how the body reacts based in part on the genetic make up of a person. Some people recover after a week from an outpatient excision of a small cancerous lesion, or up to a year if there is an extensive excision coupled with chemotherapy. It is essential to consult and connect with the primary care provider during the entire course of the treatment. Always ask question when in doubt and acquire knowledge about things that are not understood clearly.

Chapter 7 Shingles Lesions: Intervention, Treatment, Care and Recovery

Shingles

Shingles is otherwise known as Herpes Zoster. It is caused by a varicella virus that also causes chicken pox. Viruses are organisms that are hard to destroy once inside the human body. They multiplies as they produces symptoms. Research has shown that viruses don't thrive well outside the human body.

Chicken pox is a disease that usually occurs during childhood. It is usually resolved, but the varicella virus still remains in the body and becomes dormant. It can be reactivated to produce herpes zoster or shingles when the immune system is either compromised or depressed. Some causative factors such as stress, fatigue, radiation, chemotherapy, steroids, aging and HIV / AIDS trigger the reactivation of the varicella zoster virus.

Varicella zoster is also infectious to people who didn't have any history of chickenpox. It is transmitted through an airborne route or by direct contact.

The Mechanism of Shingles

When the varicella virus is reactivated or is acquired, it follows a nerve pathway called dermatomes. The most common occurrences of shingles are in the chest and the back. Upon reactivation, some people with the virus will initially experience some body malaise, headache and fever. Some people will immediately feel pain such as a burning sensation, paresthesia and a needle and pinlike sensation. The occurrence of the initial symptoms are referred to as the prodromal stage of shingles. After 3 to 6 days, rashes will appear and later become vesicles filled with serous exudates. Itching is either felt before or accompanied with the rashes. Sometime during the third week or later, the vesicles are reabsorbed and turned into crusts that fall off. Skin scarring and discoloration occurs then. There are instances when painful sensation lingers after the shingles crusts fall off. This is known as postherpetic neuralgia. The appearance of symptoms and the period of healing vary substantially from one person to another.

Intervention and Treatment of Shingles

It is hard to detect shingles during the prodromal stage because of the absence of skin rashes. Most people experience headache, body malaise and fever attributed to other type of diseases. Some people remain asymptomatic until the rash appears. An antiviral drug called acyclovir is usually prescribed. The drug is more effective if administered during the early stages during the initial appearance of rashes. Delayed administration may result in postherpetic neuralgia. Anti-pain medications or analgesics are prescribed depending on the persons' pain tolerance.

Caring and Recovering after Shingles

For some people with postherpetic neuralgia, the pain seems to be never ending. A stronger analgesic may be prescribed. The areas where crusts have fallen off may produce discoloration and scars. It can be embarrassing for some people especially if the scars cannot be hidden under clothing.

Eating a well balanced diet will help in resolving scars. There is a possibility of another breakout in the future if the immune system is compromised or some causative factor triggers it. Shingles is a threatening disease for older adults. A vaccine called zostavax may be administered and prescribed by a physician to reduce the likelihood of outbreaks in older adults, aged 50 years and above.

Chapter 8 Pressure Ulcer Lesions and Wounds: Intervention, Treatment, Care and Recovery

Pressure Ulcer

A pressure ulcer is defined as a localized injury to a specific area where there is soft tissue overlying a bone. It is also known as bedsore and decubitus ulcer. It occurs mostly on the bony prominences such as heels, hips, sacrum and coccyx area. The sacrum is the vertebral bone at the base of the spine while the coccyx is a bone at the end of the spine. A pressure ulcer may also occur in other parts of the body such as back of the head, elbows, knees and ankles.

Causative Factors of Pressure Ulcer

There are numerous factors that can give rise to a pressure ulcer. The common causes are immobility, aging, malnutrition, external forces like shearing and friction and obstructive diseases of the circulatory system. Immobility implies staying in the same position for longer periods of time that could be from an hour to a day. It usually occurs with bed-ridden people. Their inability to move due to certain diseases of the skeletal, muscular and nervous system predisposes them to pressure ulcers. The pressure that is exerted on the soft tissue overlying a bone such as in the hips in a side lying position causes collapse of the capillaries leading to the death of the tissue. It is otherwise known as tissue necrosis. Once tissue necrosis occurs, the initial stage of pressure ulcer appears.

Aging and its process renders the epidermal layer of the skin thinner and less elastic. This process results in the vulnerability of the older adults to pressure ulcers. Recovery for them is slow primary because of reduced blood flow and the degeneration of blood vessels. There has been reports about higher incidents of pressure ulcers in nursing homes. Different managerial techniques have been implemented to monitor and prevent pressure ulcers from occurring in nursing homes.

Malnutrition is the insufficient intake of necessary nutrients needed by a healthy body. Protein is the building block of the cellular process as it is the main ingredient for cellular development. Protein deficiency renders the soft tissues overlying a bone weaker and less tolerant of pressure. Albumin, a required protein in bodily processes, can be checked through laboratory testing. Greater than 3.5 g/dl is good for older adults. A well balanced diet is always desirable with food intake containing the recommended daily allowances of vitamins and minerals, carbohydrates, fats and proteins. Drinking 6 -9 glasses of water on a daily basis also helps with metabolism.

Shearing is a force that is created through sliding between surfaces. This type of force causes stretching of the skin, and the pressure that is exerted on the skin through the process renders an occlusion to the blood supply of the body part in contact. It is a combination of the sliding activity and the pressure from the body. This happens in everyday life and those people who are immobile get most of this through positioning, transfer and elevation of the head of the bed. Constant shearing eventually leads to a skin ulcer.

Friction is another type of force that occurs through the rubbing of the skin on another surface. This happens to all of us. Depending on the amount of pressure and exposure, it can cause a superficial abrasive tendency on the epidermis. If it constantly occurs to a person, the abrasion will lead to a deeper wound. The scrape of skin produced by a pair of ill-fitting shoes worn the entire day is an example of how a frictional force can cause ulcer.

Finally, there are obstructive diseases of the circulatory system. An example of these obstructive diseases is hypotension or having a low blood pressure. In hypotension, there is a decrease in the micro vascular circulation in the capillary beds of the blood vessels. It causes both insufficient oxygenation and blood pooling. The circulatory system of the human body is comprised of the heart and the blood vessels. Arteries, veins and capillaries are the blood vessels that carry the blood throughout the body. Capillaries are the smallest blood vessels of the body. They are also the place where micro vascular circulation occurs. Substances and gases are being exchanged in the capillaries. Arteries carry the oxygenated blood to the capillaries while veins carry the deoxygenated blood to the heart. Measures to elevate blood pressure such as adequate hydration and assertive movement of the body parts tend to correct the situation. There are medications prescribed for low blood pressure and an increase in salt intake can also help. In most cases, hypotension is not the leading cause of pressure ulcers.

Stages of Pressure Ulcer

There are at least 4 known stages of pressure ulcer; stages 1, 2, 3 and 4. Each of these stages have their own characteristic. If a person knows the stage, remedy through treatment is most effective. it also prevents the further aggravation of a pressure ulcer. In cases of stage 4 ulcer, a whole team of medical professionals will be treating it. Systemic infection will be the dreaded complication if treatment is not effective. Depending on what stage it is, wound healing is usually a long process particularly with older adults and the immunocompromised. Older adults continuously undergo degenerative changes in their bodies due to the aging process.

Stage 1

This stage is characterized by a reddened area in the soft tissue overlying a bony part. The skin usually returns to its normal color after some passage of time when the pressure source is removed. A good example is position changes from side lying for longer periods of time to a prone position. There is no damage to the epidermis at this time but recovery is needed before repositioning is done. Massaging the reddened area is not recommended because it furthers the damage the tissue.

Stage 2

This is a stage where the superficial skin or epidermis is missing. It may also involve the dermis. It is a shallow type of ulceration and looks like an abrasion. It appears pink or red in color and there is presence of some blisters. It can be treated with a quick dressing. Tight shoes have abrasive tendencies. The combination of some or all of the causative factors mentioned above may cause a pressure ulcer at this stage.

Stage 3

This stage involves the epidermis all the way down to the subcutaneous tissue of a body part. The color may be related to the underlying tissue. Color varies from red to white. It appears like a deep crater with or without exudates or drainage. Exudates are liquid like materials consisting of substances derived from the inflammatory process. Healing in this stage will entail a longer period of time. Infection is very common particularly if the wound is not covered.

Stage 4

This is the ultimate and final stage of a pressure ulcer wherein it extends to the muscles and bones. There is massive destruction of tissues. It appears to be covered with some sloughed skin. The color can be a combination of some yellowish slough material and a pinkish to reddish tissue color with some whiteness. Healing may take months to years depending on a person's situation. Immobility and poor nutritional intake prolongs the healing period. This is the stage where the members of a multidisciplinary healthcare team work hard to prevent infection and promote wound healing.

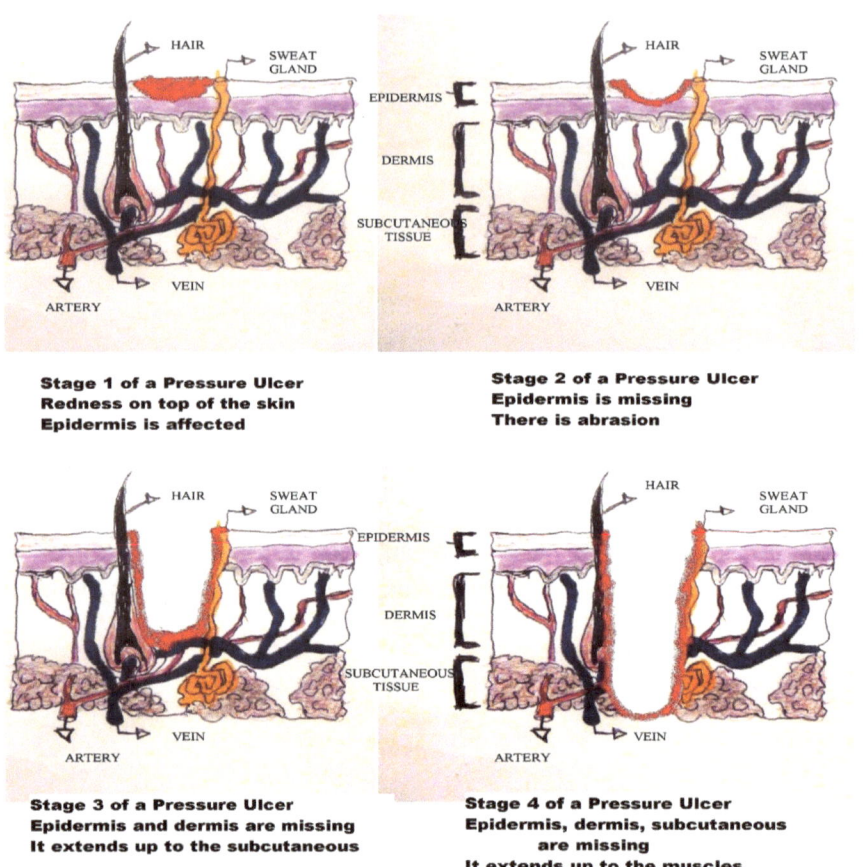

Stage 1 of a Pressure Ulcer
Redness on top of the skin
Epidermis is affected

Stage 2 of a Pressure Ulcer
Epidermis is missing
There is abrasion

Stage 3 of a Pressure Ulcer
Epidermis and dermis are missing
It extends up to the subcutaneous

Stage 4 of a Pressure Ulcer
Epidermis, dermis, subcutaneous
are missing
It extends up to the muscles

Recently, researchers have added "unstageable pressure ulcer". This type of ulcer is characterized by a deep crater and the presence of black eschar. A deep crater is a depressed area that extends up to the bone. This crater ends with a black eschar. An eschar is a dead tissue. Eschar forms because of the lack of blood supply as well as the absence of cellular nutrients. This pressure ulcer is considered unstageable because the eschar covers the true depth of the ulcer.

Intervention and Treatment for the Stages of Pressure Ulcer

In stage 1, removal and modification of the causative factor is the main goal. This can be achieved through the reduction of sliding and shearing forces. An overhead trapeze is beneficial for some immobile people as it allows them to actively use their upper extremities. Mobility through ambulation and exercises enables tissue perfusion. Exercises may be performed with a full range of motion depending on the physical ability of the person. Adequate hydration and an improved nutritional intake will also increase tissue perfusion. In this stage, never massage the affected area to prevent further tissue damage.

For stage 2 pressure ulcers; removing the causative factor, adequate hydration, nutritional intake and wound care are the essentials. A cleansing solution such as saline is used during wound care. Antiseptic solution is not used because it hinders the healing of the ulcer. Moisture is essential to promote the growth of the new epidermal tissue of the skin. Refer to the wound care management section of this book.

For Stage 3 and Stage 4, the treatment entails a great deal of work. On top of the care measures mentioned from stages 1 & 2, debridement and constant dressing changes are needed. Debridement is a process of removing a dead and necrotic tissue. This is to promote the formation of a new tissue. The types of debridement that are commonly used are mechanical, autolytic, chemical and surgical. Mechanical debridement utilizes wet to dry dressing changes. This debridement requires the application of a wet dressing before a dry one. An autolytic debridement is a type of debridement where a persons' own enzymes perform the work of debridement. It does ordinarily not occur in infected wounds. Chemical debridement utilizes specific chemical compounds such as chemical enzymes to do the process of debridement. This is primarily beneficial when mechanical debridement is not an option. Finally, surgical debridement utilizes surgical instruments such as a scalpel to remove the necrotic tissue. This is done when there is a large amount of necrotic tissue and when speed is a requirement.

There are instances when an infection occurs during debridement. A culture or a specimen from the wound exudate is acquired to determine the infectious agent. It is sent to the laboratory for analysis. Trained nurses and medical professionals are the main caretakers of the person with stages 2 to 4 pressure ulcer.

Care and Recovery from Pressure Ulcer

Recovering from stages 3 and 4 of a pressure ulcer can take longer. The causative factors must be considered carefully. When experienced and well trained caregivers and medical personnel do the care management, motivation and self-care will lessen the period of healing. Assessing the wound site every day for signs of infection, eating a well balanced diet, maintaining adequate tissue oxygenation through exercises and adherence to the care plan are the basic foundation for enhancing wound healing. After some time after healing of the wound site was achieved, recurrence of pressure ulcer may happen. Preventing pressure ulcers through constant movement and nutritional intake is the key.

Chapter 9 : Burn Lesions and Wounds: Intervention, Treatment, Care and Recovery

Burns

Burns are a difficult subject to discuss. There are a lot of concepts involved. It requires a lengthy discussion involving the areas of care and treatment. This chapter is presented to provide the reader with the necessary basic understanding of the subject.

A burn is defined as an injury to the skin and its structure caused by thermal, chemical, radiation or electrical means. The existence of burned skin is primarily the result of accidents. Mishandling and unintentional contact is the usual cause. The extent or degree of the burned skin depends on the amount of force of the contact and the longevity of the accident.

During the time when a burn is occurring, the sensation of pain signals the affected person to withdraw from the source. The sensation is brought about by the nerves that are being destroyed in the process. A quick response of withdrawing from the source limits the extent of damage to the skin. A series of inflammatory body responses occur after an episode.

The total body surface that was burned can be estimated using the Rule of 9. This rule implies that face constitutes 9 %, each of upper extremities is 9 %, each of the lower extremities is 18 %, genitalia is 1 %, the whole chest including the abdomen is 18 % and the whole back is 18 %.

Causes of Burns

The causes of burns are directly related to the source. Thermal burns occur when the skin is exposed to heat from liquids, hot objects and flames of fire. Chemical burns are caused by the strong acid in certain chemicals such as sulfuric acid. Burns from radiation are usually caused by ultraviolet rays from the sun and tanning beds. Electrical burns are caused by mishandling of electrical appliances such as from a broken prong of a plug in an electrical outlet. The degree of the burned area can extend up to the dermis and in rare cases to muscles and bones.

Types of Burn According to the Area Involved

First Degree Burns

This type of burn is also known as superficial and partial thickness burn. The burned area is confined to the top of the skin specifically the epidermis. It appears red, dry and painful. Some nerves are also involved causing painful sensation.

Second Degree Burns

This type of burn is also known as deep partial thickness. It extends up to the dermis and possibly the subcutaneous tissue. It appears red, swollen, moist and with painful vesicles.

Third Degree Burns

This is a full thickness burns that extends up to the subcutaneous tissue. It appears as pearly white, dry and leathery skin. There is no pain because the nerves are burned.

Fourth Degree Burns

This type of burn extends up to the muscles and even the bones. It appears as charred black, dry and painless.

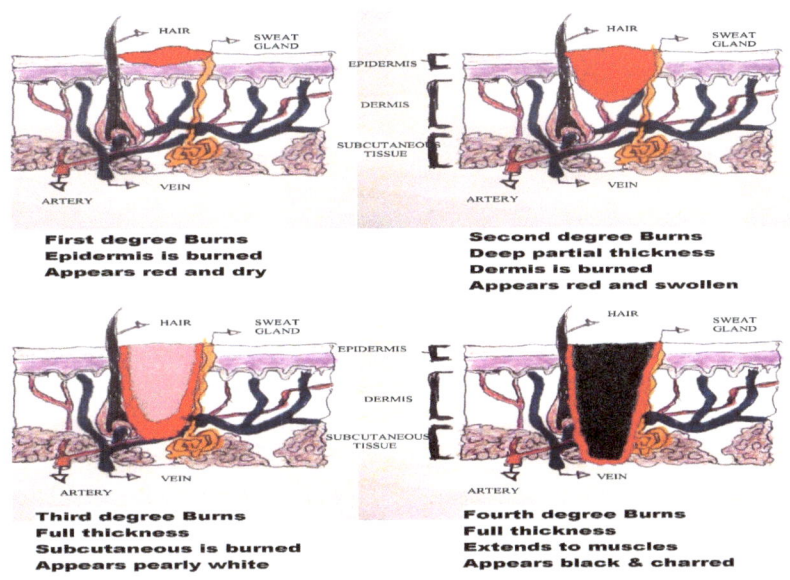

Bodily Response During a Burn Episode / Pathophysiology of Burns

The initial reaction of the body to burns is an inflammatory response. For larger burned areas such as in third and fourth degree burns, the inflammatory response is systemic. The body tries to maintain homeostasis and bodily equilibrium. A typical inflammatory response consists of histamine release, dilation of blood vessels, swelling and neural responses. Histamines are neurotransmitters that are initially released during a burn episode. Through their release, the inflammatory process is triggered. Histamines are composed of nitrogen compounds that act to transmit neural responses. Blood vessels dilate as part of the histamine release. The dilation causes the redness of the burned area.

The blood vessels also become permeable causing the release of plasma proteins and body fluid to the affected part. This results in swelling. Pain receptors like bradykinin are released in the process. This causes painful sensations. White blood cells are also released to combat infectious agents through phagocytosis and phinocytosis. Phagocytosis is the process where white blood cells engulf a pathogen such as bacteria. Phinocytosis is the process where white blood cells drink the pathogens. Neurotransmitters such catecholamines are released causing an increase in the heart rate and vascular resistance. Catecholamines are neurotransmitters of the nervous system. The most abundant of these neurotransmitters are epinephrine (also called adrenaline), dopamine and norepinephrine.

The fluid from the body shifts and is lost during an extensive burn episode. This shift causes a decrease in the circulating blood volume. Fluid leakage occurs in the first 24 hours causing a drop in the blood pressure. Electrolytes in the body are also affected by the initial fluid shift causing hyperkalemia (an increase in potassium level) and hyponatremia (a decrease in sodium level). Furthermore the death of cells occurs resulting in hemolysis of red blood cells and an elevated hematocrit. Hemolysis means the destruction of blood cells while hematocrit is the volume percentage of red blood cells in the blood.

The ability to regulate temperature is reduced because of the skin loss. Receptors for regulating temperature are present in the skin. Major burn episodes impair the regulatory process. Burn trauma also cause paralytic ileus and Curling's ulcer. Paralytic ileus is the absence of movement in the intestines while Curling's ulcer is erosion in some parts of the intestines. Since there is fluid loss, tissue perfusion is also decreased affecting the blood flow to the kidneys. If the kidneys receive inadequate blood supply, acute renal failure occurs. Finally, metabolic acidosis prevails due to loss of bicarbonates. The acid base balance is regulated by both bicarbonates and acids. Metabolic acidosis is a condition where the amount of acid in the body is excessive. Kidney failure in a burn episode is the common cause of acidosis because the kidneys are not able to remove sufficient amounts of acid.

Interventions and Treatment

For minor burns, eliminating the source and stopping the exposure is the initial step. If clothing is affected, drop to the ground and roll to put out the flames. Run the affected part in cool tap water through the faucet or the shower. Apply a prescribed antibiotic solution to the burned area if necessary. Cover with a non-adherent dressing to prevent infection. Analgesic or pain relievers can be administered if pain is severe.

In cases of second to fourth degree burns, a more comprehensive intervention is needed. Stabilizing the vital signs is the primary goal. Airway clearance and gas exchange need to be ensured to enable tissue perfusion. Since there is fluid loss, fluid replacement is administered. Either colloids such as whole blood or electrolytes are used in fluid replacement.

Temperature regulation is impaired exposing the burned person to chilling and hypothermia. Room temperature must be adjusted and drafts avoided. Infection is a major complication for bigger burned areas. Aseptic technique in changing wound dressing is necessary. The administration of a prescribed antibacterial solution is also necessary to prevent infection. Silvadene, silver nitrate or sulfamylon are some of the commonly prescribed antibiotics. Debridement is done to remove the necrotic tissue. This method is somewhat similar to the debridement for pressure ulcers.

Skin grafts maybe ordered to cover the wounded area. They also become a part of the new skin. Some types of skin grafts include autografts or skin from the burned person, homografts that are skin from another person, heterografts that are skin from animals, and synthetic skin substitutes.

The pain that is experience in an extensive burn is so intense that greater doses of analgesics are required. Morphine is usually the analgesic that is prescribed. Anti-anxiety drugs such as ativan are also prescribed to alleviate anxiety or panic attacks.

Nutritional intake is very important because of bodily trauma. The body needs nutrients for wound healing and stabilization. Amino acid is the component of protein in any food that enables formation of new tissue. A total parenteral nutrition may also be ordered for an extensively burned person.

Care and Recovery After A Burn Episode

Rehabilitation is a difficult process. Depending on the location of the burned part, physical image is affected. The application of a skin graft enables the burned person to face the public with confidence. Much of recovery is aimed at total body functioning. Activities are emphasized to promote optimization of movement, prevention of contractures and adaptation to activities of daily living. Both occupational and physical therapy are needed in the rehabilitation process. A well balanced diet is also necessary to sustain recovery.

Glossary

Analgesic = is a type of drug that removes the sensation of pain. It is usually available over the counter but narcotics such as morphine require a prescription.

Antiseptic = is a solution that has the ability to eliminate microbes. It is usually made up of strong chemicals that kill bacteria and other microorganisms.

Aseptic technique =is a method used to ensure that there is no microbial contamination. Washing hands and using gloves are parts of the aseptic technique.

Catecholamines = are substances in the body that help in the transmission of signals from the nervous system. They stimulate various organs of the body making bodily processes become faster. The most common catecholamines are adrenaline and dopamine.

Debridement = is a procedure of removing dead tissue in a wound. It is achieved through methods such as mechanical, surgical, chemical and autolyis.

Dermatome = is an area of the skin that is supplied by a single spinal nerve root. It is also known as a nerve pathway.

Erythema = is the reddish discoloration of the skin because of the excessive concentration of blood within the blood vessels. It commonly exists in inflammatory conditions such as in a burn episode.

Eschar = is a dead tissue on top of a wound. It is usually black in color. It is removed during debridement. Underneath the eschar is a new tissue.

Exudate = is a fluid or a drainage that rises out from a cell or an organ. Wound exudates are usually related to an infectious process.

Granulation tissue = is a new form of a connective tissue that grows during the healing of a wound. Care is taken during dressing changes so as not to destroy this new tissue.

Histamines = is a specific compound in the body that produces inflammatory responses. Sneezing and phlegm formation during an allergy attack is an example of a histamine reaction.

Hyponatremia = is a condition where there is low sodium in the body. The standard laboratory value for sodium is 135 − 145 mEq/L.

Hyperkalemia = is a condition where there is excess potassium in the body. The standard laboratory value for potassium is 3.5 − 5.0 mEq/L.

Hypovolemic shock = is a condition where there is a decrease in the amount of blood circulating in the body. When this happens, there is insufficient oxygenation of the bodily tissues. This condition is a medical emergency and can lead to death.

Homeostasis = is a state wherein the human body maintains an environment where the functionality of the various systems are stabilized. The indicators of homeostasis are the vital signs.

Paresthesia = is a sensation of numbness, tingling or pricking. It is commonly referred to as sensations of needles and pins.

Phagocytosis = is a mechanism of eating or engulfing foreign substances such as bacteria. It is primarily a function of the white blood cells in the body. It occurs during an inflammatory response and when there is an infection.

Prodromal Stage = is a stage in the disease process wherein a number of symptoms exists. The symptoms are not specific and severe. This is the stage where it is difficult to diagnose a specific condition and laboratory work is necessary to confirm a diagnosis.

Postherpetic Neuralgia = is a condition where there is severe pain along the nerve pathways cause by the varicella zoster virus. It is a lingering pain after the rashes of the shingles have gone away.

Skin grafts = is a transplanted skin cover that is intended to facilitate the formation of new tissue. It is put in place during the process of wound healing. It is also used for cosmetic purposes where scars are hard to remove.

Vasodilation = is a condition where the blood vessels become dilated or widened. It is due to the relaxation of the smooth muscles in the walls of the blood vessels.

Vital signs = are indicators and parameters of the condition of the human body in various states. They comprise respiratory rate, blood pressure, pulse rate and temperature.

Wound dressing = is a piece of gauze pad that is used in covering up a wounded area of the human body. There had been variations in the production of wound dressing during the past years such that hydrocolloids, hydrogels, transparent films, foams and alginates are options that can be used for dressing a particular wound.

References

I would like to express my gratitude to:

Dr. Lee Robbins for his support in writing this book.

Anatomy and Physiology, Wiley and Sons, New Jersey, 2007
Fundamentals of Nursing 7th Edition, Mosby, Canada, 2009
Gerontological Nursing 2nd Edition, ANCC, Maryland, 2009
Medical – Surgical Nursing 4th Edition, Prentice Hall, New Jersey, 2008
NCLEX PN, Saunders, Missouri, 2003
NCLEX RN, Mosby, Missouri, 1999
Nursing Assistants, Mosby, Philadelphia, 2004
Nursing Interventions and Clinical Skills, Mosby, Missouri, 2004
Nursing Procedures and Protocols, Lippincott, Philadelphia 2003
Pathophysiology of Disease 2nd Edition, Appleton and Lange, 1997
Pharmacology in Nursing 21st Edition, Mosby, Missouri 2001
Principles and Practice of Psychiatric Nursing 6th edition, Mosby, Missouri 1998
The Johns Hopkins Consumer Guide to Medical Tests, Medletter Associates Inc, New York, 2001
The Johns Hopkins White Papers, Hypertension and Stroke, Medletter Associates Inc, New York, 2003
Wikipidea Free Internet Dictionary

Index

abrasion, 10, 16, 17, 34, 35
Acetic acid, 22
Acne vulgaris, 14
alcoholism, 24
analgesic, 32, 41
antibacterial, 22, 41
antibiotic solution, 22, 41
antibiotics, 13, 14, 24, 41
antimicrobial, 22
antiseptic, 22, 23, 24
arsenic compounds, 25
Arterial blood, 20
Aseptic technique, 41, 42
asymmetrical, 25, 27
asymptomatic, 13, 25, 32
Athlete's foot, 15
autografts, 41
autolytic debridement, 37
Basal cell carcinoma, 26
bedsore, 33
benzoyl peroxide, 14
bicarbonates, 40
blood, 9, 12, 13, 15, 17, 18, 19, 20, 25,
    26, 27, 33, 34, 36, 40, 41, 42, 43
blood loss, 20
body malaise, 31, 32
bruising, 16
bulla, 15
Burns, 1, 7, 8, 13, 38, 40
catecholamines, 40, 42
Cellulitis, 13
Chemical burns, 38
Chemical debridement, 37
chemical enzymes, 37
chemotherapy, 13, 28, 29, 30, 31
chicken pox, 31
cisplatin, 29
clot, 18, 20
coccyx, 33
Collagen, 18, 24

comedones, 14
crusts, 15, 23, 31, 32
cryosurgery, 28, 29
Curling's ulcer, 40
Dandruffs, 15
debridement, 13, 14, 23, 37, 41, 42
decubitus ulcer, 33
Dermatofibroma, 15
dermatologist, 12, 25, 27
dermis, 4, 9, 13, 15, 18, 35, 38, 39
direct pressure, 20
dressing, 14, 20, 21, 23, 24, 29, 35, 37,
    41, 42, 43
dry gauze, 23
dryness, 14
Duoderm, 23
eczema, 14
Electrical burns, 38
enzymes, 37
epidermis, 4, 9, 12, 15, 17, 27, 34, 35, 39
epinephrine, 40
epithelial cell, 27
Epithelialization, 18
erosions, 15
eschar, 36, 42
excision, 28, 30
Excisional biopsy, 28
fever, 19, 24, 31, 32
First Degree Burns, 39
fissures, 15
fluorouracil, 29
forceps, 22, 23
Fourth Degree Burns, 39
Freckles, 15
Friction, 34
Gauze dressing, 23
gauze pad, 22, 28, 43
granular tissue, 22, 23
granulation, 17, 18
hand gloves, 13, 22

headache, 31, 32
Healing by first intention, 17
Healing by second intention, 17
Healing by third intention, 17
hematocrit, 40
hemoglobin, 11
Hemolysis, 40
hemorrhage, 20, 21
herpes zoster, 15, 31
Herpes Zoster, 13, 31
heterografts, 41
Histamines, 40, 42
homeostasis, 40, 43
homografts, 41
Hydrocolloid, 23
hydrogel dressings, 23
Hydrogen peroxide, 22
hyperkalemia, 40
Hypertrophic scars, 18
hyponatremia, 40
Hypovolemic shock, 20, 43
imiquimod, 29
Immobility, 5, 33, 35
impetigo, 15
infection, 4, 5, 13, 15, 17, 19, 20, 21, 23, 24, 28, 29, 34, 35, 37, 41, 43
inflammatory phase, 17
inflammatory process, 24, 35, 40
inflammatory response, 24, 40, 43
itchiness, 14
laceration, 16
leukocytes, 24
liquid nitrogen, 29
macules, 4, 15
malignant lesion, 25
malnutrition, 17, 18, 24, 33
Mechanical debridement, 37
melanin, 11, 27
Melanoma, 7, 27
Metabolic acidosis, 40
Metastasis, 25, 26
migratory phase, 18
moles, 15, 27
neurotransmitters, 40
nodules, 4, 14, 15
non-adherent dressing, 4, 20, 21, 22, 41

Normal saline, 22
pain, 5, 9, 13, 14, 16, 19, 20, 23, 24, 25, 27, 31, 32, 38, 39, 41, 42, 43
papules, 4, 14, 15
Paralytic ileus, 40
paresthesia, 31
phagocytosis, 17, 40
Phagocytosis, 40, 43
Phinocytosis, 40
physical therapy, 41
pigmented nevi, 15
pinlike sensation, 31
plaque, 15
plaques, 15
postherpetic neuralgia, 31, 32
Povidone Iodine, 22
pressure ulcer, 5, 13, 15, 33, 34, 35, 36, 37
Pressure ulcer, 13
Proliferative phase, 18
protein, 24, 33, 41
Pseudomonas aeruginosa, 22
psoriasis, 14
punch biopsy, 28
purulent drainage, 19, 24
pustules, 4, 14, 15
radiation, 13, 28, 29, 30, 31, 38
radioactive substances, 29
reddened area, 35
redness, 13, 17, 29, 40
Rule of 9, 38
sacrum, 33
Saline solution, 24
scales, 14, 15
scar tissue formation, 18
scars, 18, 32, 43
seborrheic dermatitis, 14
Second Degree Burns, 39
serous exudates, 31
shave biopsy, 28
Shearing, 33
Shingles, 1, 7, 13, 31, 32
Silvadene, 41
silver nitrate, 41
skin, 4, 5, 9, 10, 11, 12, 13, 14, 15, 16, 17, 18, 19, 20, 23, 25, 26, 27, 28, 29,

32, 33, 34, 35, 37, 38, 39, 40, 41, 42, 43
Skin biopsy, 28
skin cancer, 4, 11, 25, 26, 27, 28
Skin cancer, 13, 25
skin graft, 28
skin integrity, 4, 12
skin lesion, 4, 15, 27, 28, 29
skin sample, 25, 28
sliding, 33, 36
smoking, 24
Sodium hypochloride, 22
Squamous cell carcinoma, 27
sterile, 23
Stratum basale, 9
Stratum corneum, 9
Stratum lucidum, 9
stratum spinosum, 9
sulfamylon, 41
sunscreen lotion, 26
surgery, 13, 28, 29
surgical debridement, 37
swelling, 13, 14, 16, 19, 24, 28, 29, 40
Telfa, 23

Thermal burns, 38
Third Degree Burns, 39
tissue necrosis, 33
tissue oxygenation, 24, 37
tissue perfusion, 36, 40, 41
titanium dioxide, 26
tumors, 15
ulcers, 5, 9, 12, 13, 15, 29, 33, 34, 37, 41
ultraviolet radiation, 25, 26
Varicella zoster, 31
Venous blood, 20
vesicles, 4, 13, 15, 31, 39
vitamin C, 24
Warts, 15
Wet dressings, 23
wheals, 15
wound, 4, 9, 13, 15, 16, 17, 18, 19, 20, 21, 22, 23, 24, 28, 29, 34, 35, 37, 41, 42, 43
wound care, 4, 21, 22, 23, 29, 37
wound drainage, 24
Wound irrigation, 24
zinc oxide, 26
zostavax, 32

***Kindly write a review about this book to help other readers that could benefit from this text. Thank you.

And please feel free to browse my other books @ Amazon.com

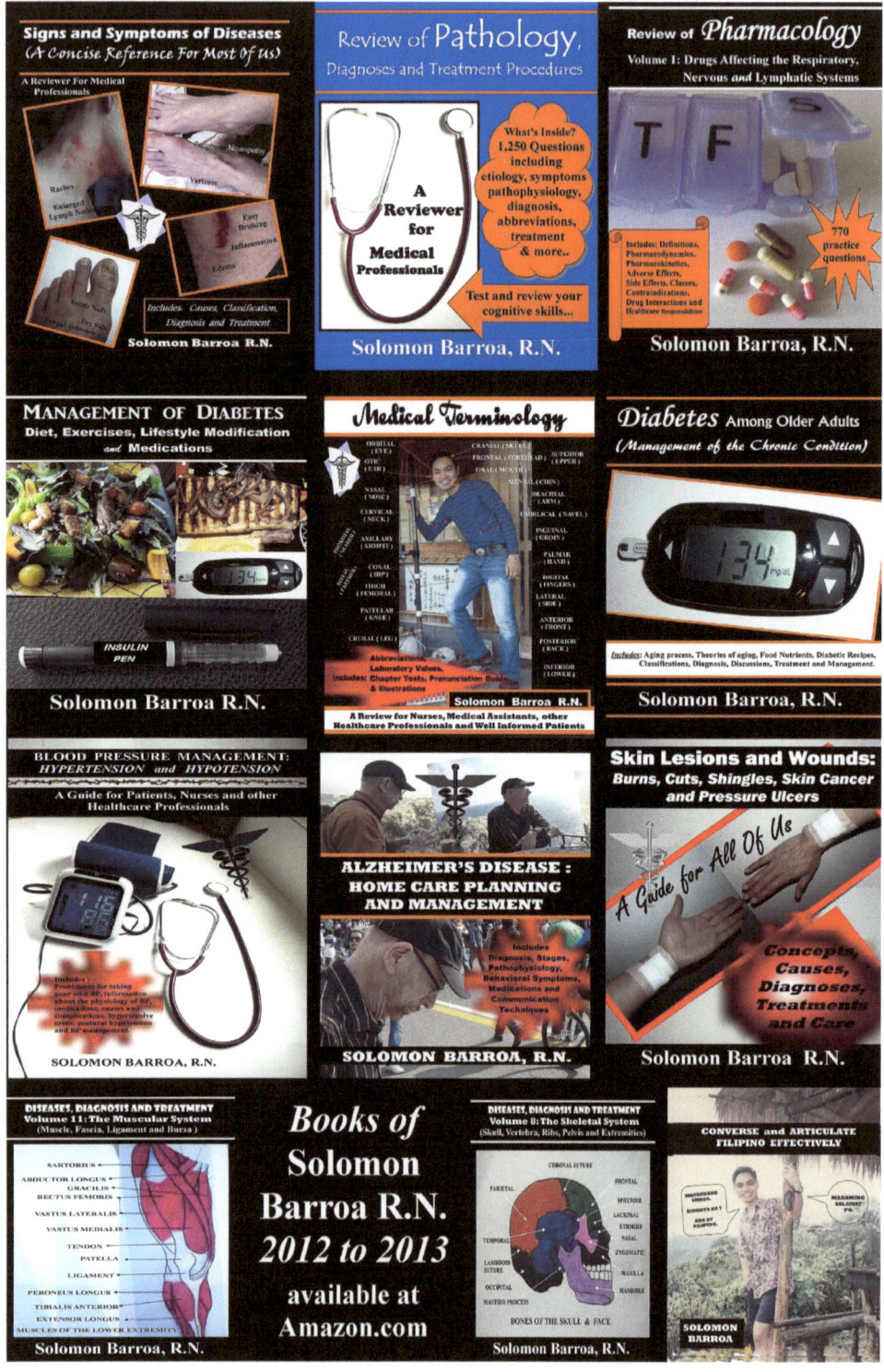

Connect with me online :

Facebook: http://www.facebook.com/solomon.barroa
Twitter: https://twitter.com/solomonbarroa
Amazon: amazon.com/author/solomonbarroa
LinkedIn: http://www.linkedin.com/in/solomonbarroa